Sensei Self Development

Mental Health Chronicles Series

Combating Negative Self-Talk

Sensei Paul David

Copyright Page

Sensei Self Development -
Combating Negative Self-Talk,
by Sensei Paul David

Copyright © 2024

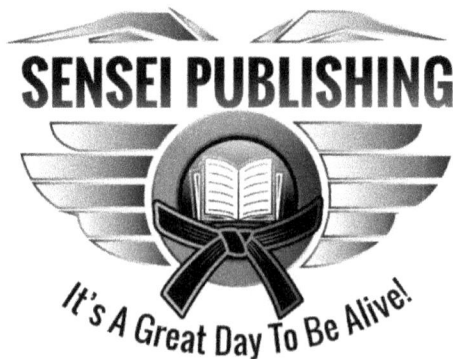

SENSEI PUBLISHING

It's A Great Day To Be Alive!

www.senseipublishing.com

@senseipublishing
senseipublishing

Get/Share Your FREE SSD Mental Health Chronicles at
www.senseiselfdevelopment.care

or

CLICK HERE

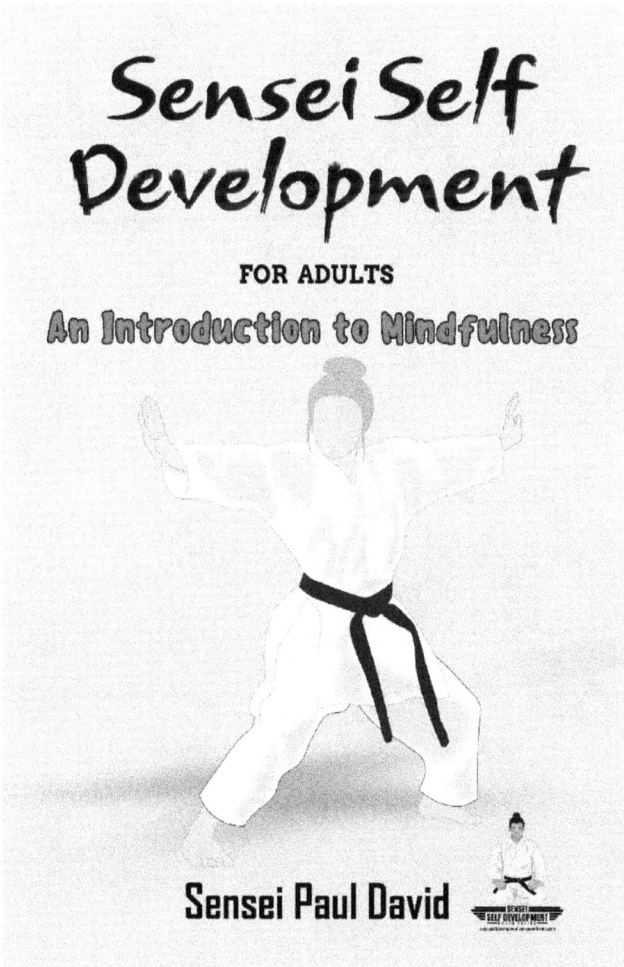

Check Out The SSD Chronicles Series CLICK HERE

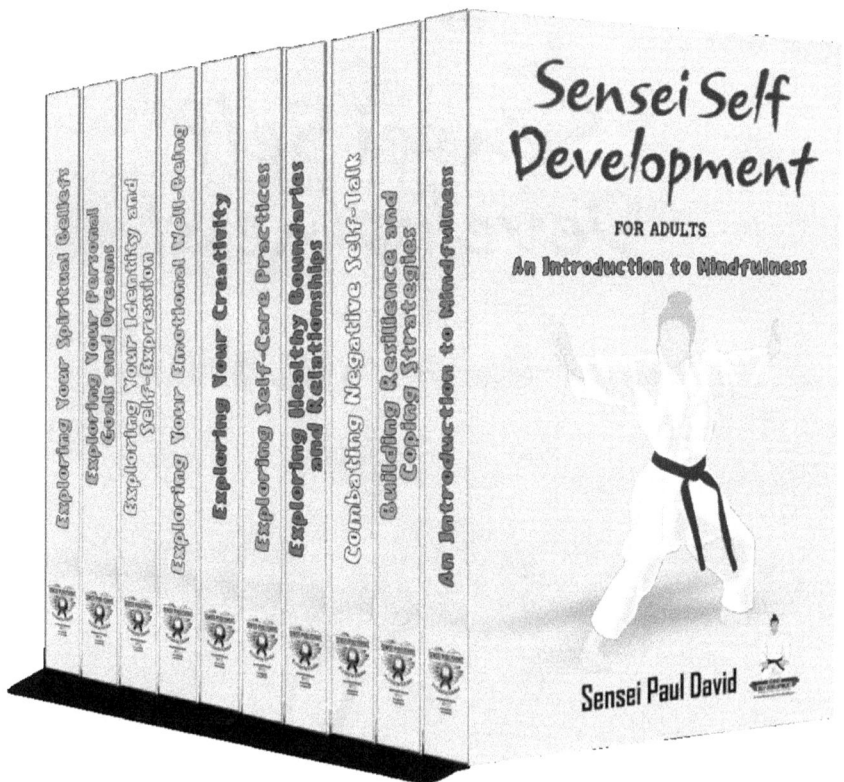

Exploring Your Spiritual Beliefs

Exploring Your Personal Goals and Dreams

Exploring Your Identity and Self-Expression

Exploring Your Emotional Well-Being

Exploring Your Creativity

Exploring Self-Care Practices

Exploring Healthy Boundaries and Relationships

Combatting Negative Self-Talk

Building Resilience and Coping Strategies

An Introduction to Mindfulness

Sensei Self Development

FOR ADULTS

An Introduction to Mindfulness

Sensei Paul David

Dedication

To those who courageously take action towards self-improvement - you are helping to evolve the world for generations to come.

- It's a great day to be alive!

If Found Please Contact:

_____

Reward If Found:

_____

MY
COMMITMENT

I, _____

commit to writing This Sensei Self
Development Journal for at least 10 days in a
row, starting: _____

Writing this journal is valuable to me because:

_____

_____

_____

_____

_____

_____

If I finish a minimum of 10 consecutive days of
writing in this journal, I will reward myself by:

_____

_____

_____

_____

_____

_____

If I don't finish 10 days of writing this journal, I will promise to:

_____

_____

_____

_____

_____

I will do the following things to ensure that I write in my Sensei Self Development Journal every day:

_____

_____

_____

_____

_____

_____

Get/Share Your FREE All-Ages Mental Health eBook Now at

www.senseiselfdevelopment.com

Or CLICK HERE

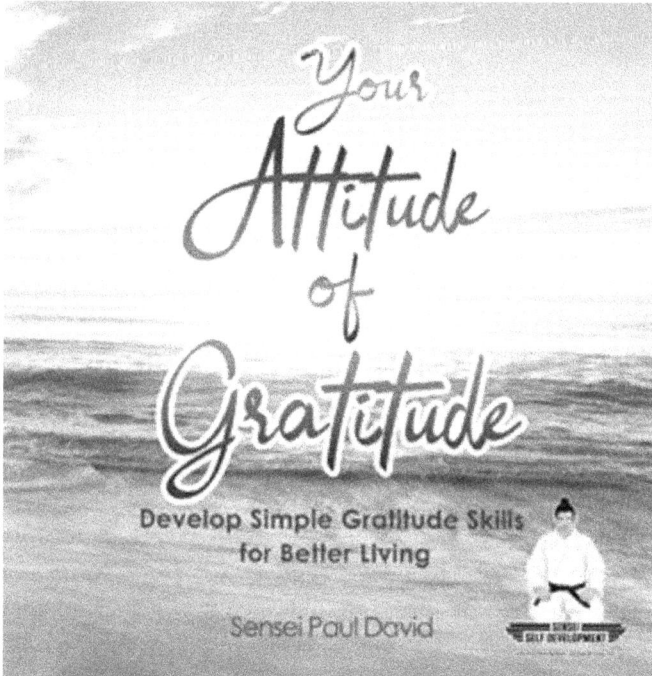

senseiselfdevelopment.com

Check Out Another Book In The
SSD BOOK SERIES:

senseipublishing.com/SSD_SERIES

CLICK HERE

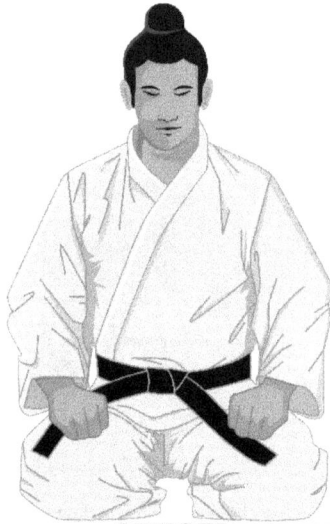

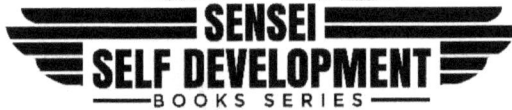

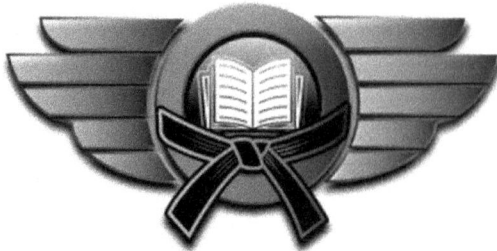

Join Our Publishing Journey!

If you would like to receive FUTURE FREE BOOKS and get to know us better, please click www.senseipublishing.com and join our newsletter by entering your email address in the pop-up box.

Follow Our Blog: senseipauldavid.ca

Follow/Like/Subscribe: Facebook, Instagram, YouTube: @senseipublishing

Scan the QR Code with your phone or tablet

to follow us on social media: Like / Subscribe / Follow

A Message From The Author:
Sensei Paul David

Dear Reader,

Welcome to the world of mental health journaling – a sacred space for self-reflection, growth, and healing. Within these pages, you hold the power to uplift your spirit, invigorate your mind, and nourish your goals.

In a world that often moves at blink-and-you'll-miss-it speed, it's crucial to make time for self-care and self-discovery.

Anxiety, stress, and emotional turbulence may have clouded your mind, making it difficult to find clarity and peace within. But fear not! Together, we will navigate the labyrinth of emotions, and experiences, helping to simplify the path to mental well-being.

This journal is not merely a bunch of blank pages awaiting your words. It is your compassionate companion, offering solace and understanding during your unique journey. Here, you are free to unburden yourself, celebrate small and large victories, and confront the challenges that may still linger.

Within the sheltered realm of these pages, there is no judgment, no expectation, and no pressure. Your unique experience and perspective hold immeasurable worth, and your voice deserves to be heard. Whether you choose to fill the lines with eloquence or simply scribble fragments of your thoughts, please remember each entry is a valuable contribution to your growth.

In this sacred space, you are challenged to take off the mask we so often wear in the outside world. It is here that you can be raw, vulnerable, and authentic – allowing your true self to be seen and embraced without reservation. By giving yourself permission to explore the depths of your emotions and confront the shadows that may lurk within, you will discover profound insights and find the healing you seek over time.

As you embark on this journaling journey, I encourage you to embrace the process itself rather than fixate solely on the outcome. Remember, it is not about reaching a certain destination or ticking off boxes on a list of accomplishments. Rather, it is about cultivating self-awareness, fostering self-compassion, and nurturing a sense of curiosity about the intricate workings of your intelligently beautiful mind.

In the quiet moments of reflection, let your pen become a bridge between your inner world and the possibilities that lie ahead. Create a sanctuary for your thoughts, fears, triumphs, and dreams. As you pour your heart onto these pages, allow your words to be a living testament to courage, resilience, and an unwavering commitment to your own well-being.

I am honored to be a part of your journey, and I believe in your ability to navigate the twists and turns with grace and resilience. Remember, you are not alone in this – countless others have walked similar paths, faced similar challenges, and emerged stronger and wiser on the other side. You have the power to reclaim all of your untapped joy, cultivate a positive mindset that serves you, and foster a deep sense of self-love and peaceful confident. – And it will take a worth effort and time.

So, open the first page of this journal with hope, curiosity, and an open heart and open mind. Embrace the transformative power of self-reflection, and allow it to guide you towards a life of greater fulfilment and peace. Each journaling session is an opportunity to not only connect with yourself but also to rekindle the light within that sometimes flickers but never extinguishes.

Remember, the pages you are about to fill are not just a record of your journey but also a testament to your strength, resilience, and indomitable spirit. Cherish this space, invest in yourself, and let your words be an ode to the magnificent journey of becoming whole.

With great respect for your decision to evolve,

Paul

MY CONVICTION

Please circle your answers below

I am DECIDING to be patient with myself and this PROCESS each time I journal toward my improved state of mental well-being

YES   NO

"The present moment is filled with joy and happiness. If you are attentive, you will see it."

Thich Nhat Hanh

Introduction

"We're all our own worst critics." This phrase may sound cliché, but it's rooted in psychological findings. Evolutionary psychologists have identified a "negativity bias" within us, a predisposition that magnifies negative experiences over positive ones. This means we often place more importance on our flaws, mistakes, and shortcomings than on our strengths or achievements.

Dr. Aaron Beck, the father of Cognitive Behavioral Therapy, points out the dangers of self-criticism. It not only leads to repetitive negative thoughts, hindering productivity, but also triggers bodily responses that can cause chronic illness and accelerate ageing.

Despite this natural inclination towards negativity, there's reason for optimism. We can counteract this bias. By understanding and acknowledging it and challenging it, we can transform self-criticism into opportunities for learning and personal growth.

So, why are we often overly critical of ourselves? Evolution plays a key role in this.

Dr. Aaron Beck explains that our brains have developed mechanisms to monitor our thoughts and actions, allowing us to recognize mistakes. Noticing deviations from our goals or expectations, like overeating or not finishing tasks, is crucial for learning. This ability helps us distinguish good from bad actions, especially when it involves our safety or moral integrity.

However, this self-monitoring can sometimes backfire, leading to harmful rumination. For instance, overthinking an awkward interaction or fixating on a minor typo at night can trap us in unproductive cycles of negative thinking.

This kind of self-criticism can have serious consequences. It's linked to depression, anxiety, substance abuse, negative self-image, and ironically, decreased motivation and productivity. A study in the Journal of Psychotherapy Integration highlights these effects. Another study from the Personality and Social Psychology Bulletin found that self-criticism often leads to an obsession with failure.

Ironically, being too hard on ourselves for minor lapses, like not completing all tasks on a to-do list, can actually hinder our ability to complete remaining tasks, despite our brains being wired to think this way.

It's a Catch-22 indeed: our evolutionary instinct is to dwell on our failures, yet this often leads to counterproductive outcomes.

So, what's the solution to this paradox?

That's what we will talk about ahead.

Before that, let's get into some facts that you would love to know.

Fast Facts

1. Increases Stress: Negative self-talk can increase stress and anxiety, as shown in studies linking self-critical thoughts with higher cortisol levels, the stress hormone.

2. Affects Performance: Research has found that negative self-talk can impair performance

in tasks, sports, and academics by reducing focus and increasing performance anxiety.

3. Linked to Depression: There's a strong correlation between negative self-talk and depression. Persistent negative thoughts can exacerbate symptoms of depression.

4. Impacts Physical Health: Chronic negative self-talk can have detrimental effects on physical health, contributing to issues like heart disease and a weakened immune system.

5. Can Be Changed: Studies in cognitive-behavioral therapy show that negative self-talk patterns can be altered through techniques like cognitive restructuring, leading to improved mental health.

6. Neurological Effects: Negative self-talk is linked to changes in the brain, including increased activity in areas associated with stress and emotion regulation. This can reinforce negative thinking patterns.

7. Influences Eating Habits: Research suggests a connection between negative self-talk and

disordered eating behaviors, as it can impact body image and control over eating.

8. Sleep Disruption: Studies have found that negative self-talk can disrupt sleep patterns, leading to insomnia or poor sleep quality, which further impacts mental and physical health.

9. Reduces Resilience: Persistent negative self-talk can decrease an individual's resilience to life's challenges, making it harder to cope with stress and recover from setbacks.

10. Affects Relationships: It can also impact relationships, as individuals with a habit of negative self-talk may have lower self-esteem and more difficulty communicating effectively with others.

Characteristics of Negative Self-Talk

Before we can discuss different ways to deal with negative self-talk, it would be beneficial to look at some of its characteristics. If you know many of its characteristics, you can deal with it in many ways. For instance one of the characteristics of negative self-talk is incessant thoughts. Now, that can be dealt with using mindfulness. Mindfulness will allow you to dissociate yourself from your thoughts by focusing on the present and hence watch them pass by. Another characteristic is distortion of reality, which means we can use Cognitive Behavioural Therapy (CBT) because it challenges and reframes irrational thoughts.

Negative self-talk typically exhibits several key characteristics:

1. Pervasiveness: It often pervades a person's thoughts, especially in challenging situations, becoming a default response.

2. Automaticity: This self-talk is automatic and reflexive, occurring without conscious effort or awareness.

3. Distortion of Reality: It involves distorted, pessimistic views of reality, often ignoring positive aspects and focusing on negatives.

4. Excessive Criticism: The individual is overly critical of themselves, often more harshly than they would be towards others.

5. Catastrophizing: It includes a tendency to anticipate the worst possible outcomes, even

when they are unlikely.

6. All-or-Nothing Thinking: This involves seeing things in black-and-white terms, without recognizing any middle ground or gray areas.

7. Personalization: There's a tendency to take things personally and blame oneself for events that are not entirely under one's control.

8. Overgeneralization: Drawing broad, negative conclusions based on limited evidence or single events.

9. Filtering: Focusing exclusively on negative aspects of a situation, while ignoring any positive elements.

10. Mind Reading: Assuming to know what others are thinking, usually negatively, without sufficient evidence.

How to Deal with Negative Self-Talk

Cognitive Behavioral Therapy (CBT)

CBT is a practical approach to mental health, particularly effective in addressing negative self-talk.

Negative self-talk often stems from cognitive distortions, which are essentially misinterpretations of reality. These distortions can make everything seem worse than it actually is. For instance:

- All-or-Nothing Thinking: Viewing things in absolute terms, like "If I'm not perfect, I'm a failure."
- Overgeneralization: Drawing broad conclusions from a single event.
- Mental Filtering: Focusing solely on the negatives and overlooking any positives.
- Jumping to Conclusions: Predicting the worst without enough evidence to back it up.
- Should Statements: Imposing rigid expectations on yourself, often leading to disappointment.

CBT tackles these distortions through a structured process:

1. Identification: Recognizing the negative or distorted thoughts.

2. Examination: Analyzing these thoughts critically to see if they really hold up.

3. Challenging: Debating with your own thoughts to test their validity.

4. Replacement: Substituting the irrational thoughts with more balanced and realistic ones.

By consistently applying CBT techniques, you can significantly improve your mental well-being and reduce the impact of negative self-talk.

Here's an example:

Imagine you've just given a presentation at work, and it didn't go as well as you hoped. You find yourself thinking, "I totally messed up. I'm terrible at my job."

Step 1: Identification of Negative Self-Talk

- First, recognize this thought for what it is: a negative self-statement. It's an all-or-nothing statement that labels your entire performance based on one aspect.

Step 2: Examination of the Thought

- Next, examine this thought critically. Ask yourself some questions: Did everything about the presentation go poorly? Were there parts that went well? Is it true that making a mistake in a presentation means you're terrible at your job?

Step 3: Challenging the Thought

- Challenge the validity of your initial thought. Consider evidence against it: Remember times you've done well at your job, feedback from colleagues, or aspects of the presentation that were successful. Also, consider the unrealistic standard of not making any mistakes. Everyone makes mistakes; it's a part of learning and growing professionally.

Step 4: Replacement with a Balanced Thought

- Finally, replace the negative thought with a more balanced and realistic one. Instead of thinking, "I'm terrible at my job," you might say, "This presentation didn't go as well as I hoped, but I've had successful ones in the past. I can learn from this experience and improve for next time."

Through this process, you're not just dismissing the negative thought; you're examining and replacing it with a perspective that's both more accurate and more constructive. This approach can lead to a more balanced self-view, less anxiety, and a greater sense of competence and resilience.

Positive Reappraisal

Positive Reappraisal, or looking at the bright side as my psychologist friend likes to call it, is actually considered a CBT technique as well. But writing it separately would just be too much information cinched together in the CBT section. It will get lost.

Positive reappraisal is essentially playing with the meaning you assign to an event. You broke your legs. Rather than think of it as something bad. You think it's a blessing (like Bruce Lee did). Maybe you get time off and get to write a book you'd been putting off. It could be seen as an opportunity to test or build your mental fortitude. It could also be seen as a catalyst for your life – maybe if you never had your leg broken, you would never rethink your life and spend your life day in and day out, wasting it away for the success of someone else.

Some might argue this is delusional. But it is actually not – objectively speaking. As far as science is concerned, every meaning you assign to an event (good or bad) can be called delusional. Take death, for instance, you can successfully argue that death is good. If you start with the premise life is suffering and there is no suffering after you die (It's just nothingness). Then life is good (as long as you assert that absence of suffering is good). Similarly, you can argue, equally successfully, that death is bad. Hopefully, I don't have to lay that out for you. You can give me ten arguments off the top of your head.

These arguments are not delusional. They are logically coherent (meaning the conclusions follow from their premise.)

Similarly, if you have a premise that it is rational to minimize suffering and maximise wellbeing, it would make logical sense for you to view a leg break as something positive because that will alleviate suffering and increase wellbeing. If you are not doing that, you are being irrational. What's the point of viewing a leg break as negative when objectively speaking it is neither good or bad.

I am usually advised by my editors that, "David, keep it tight. Don't get into phiosophical arguments. Just show them how to do it" But I love my philosophy. So I hope you will forgive me for this excursion. Getting back to practicalities.

Here's how positive reappraisal works:

1. Identifying the Stressful Situation: First, you acknowledge the situation that is causing stress or negative emotions. For instance, let's say you're feeling overwhelmed by a new project at work.

2. Acknowledging Your Initial Reaction: Recognize how you initially perceive this situation. Perhaps you're thinking, "This is impossible; I can't handle this."

3. Searching for Positive Aspects: Next, deliberately look for positive aspects or potential benefits in the situation. Ask yourself questions like, "What can I learn from this experience?" or "How can this challenge help me grow?" In our example, you might realize

that this project is an opportunity to develop new skills or demonstrate your capabilities.

Or you might compare yourself to your neighbour, who works at a much harder job than you. Or you may think yourself lucky for actually having a job and being able to put food in front of your kids.

You can go many ways with this.

Mindfulness and Meditation

The last two strategies – CBT and Positive Reappraisal – involved engaging with the thought (challenging its contents or meaning), Mindfulness and meditation attempt to stand clear of thoughts.

Is there any point in fighting with clouds? You should just stand aside and watch them pass by. So it is with negative thoughts.

According to this line of thinking, your thoughts are not yours. They appear in your head. Have you ever had any thoughts you'd *never* endorse? Exactly! Some thoughts we endorse. Some, we would never. You know why? Because they are not us.

According to Buddha, suffering stems from identifying with these thoughts.

Rather than changing them, Meditation and mindfulness try to disassociate with thoughts so they do not influence your emotions.

And, believe it or not, this works. You have countless studies and meta-analysis published that have shown the effectiveness of both meditation and mindfulness.

Moreover, mindfulness is particularly effective against negative self-talk because it advocates living in the now. Since most of our woes are about the past or the future, staying in the present is very effective.

Here's how you can practise mindfulness:

To practice mindfulness, find a quiet and comfortable space where you can sit or lie down without distractions. Begin by setting a timer for a short period, like 5 to 10 minutes, to help maintain focus. Close your eyes and take deep, steady breaths, concentrating on the sensation of air entering and leaving your body. As thoughts come into your mind, observe them without judgment or engagement, allowing them to pass by like leaves on a stream. Whenever you notice your attention drifting away from your breath, gently guide it back, maintaining a sense of patience and kindness towards yourself. With each session, you'll grow more attuned to the present moment, fostering a sense of calm and clarity in your daily life.

Mindfulness can be seamlessly integrated into everyday life by bringing a conscious presence and awareness to your daily activities. Here's how:

1. Mindful Eating: Pay attention to the taste, texture, and aroma of your food. Eat slowly, savoring each bite, and notice how your body feels as you eat.

2. Mindful Walking: While walking, focus on the sensation of your feet touching the ground, the rhythm of your steps, and the feel of the air against your skin.

3. Mindful Listening: When someone is speaking, listen with full attention without planning your response or getting distracted by your thoughts.

4. Mindful Breathing: Throughout the day, take a few moments to focus on your breath. Notice the rise and fall of your chest and the sensation of air flowing in and out.

5. Mindful Observation: Take a few minutes to observe your surroundings or an object. Notice colors, textures, patterns, and details you usually overlook.

6. Mindful Working: Engage fully with your work tasks, bringing your full attention to each task, one at a time, without multitasking.

7. Mindful Pause: Regularly take short breaks to check in with yourself. Notice any bodily sensations, thoughts, or emotions without judgment.

Incorporating these practices into your daily routine can help you become more present and engaged in the moment, reducing stress and increasing enjoyment and effectiveness in your activities.

Meditation

Mindfulness and meditation are closely related practices, but they have distinct characteristics:

Mindfulness is a state of active, open attention to the present moment. It involves being fully aware of your thoughts, feelings, bodily sensations, and surrounding environment without judgment. Mindfulness can be practiced at any time, regardless of what you're doing. It's about tuning into the present experience rather than dwelling on the past or worrying about the future. You can practice mindfulness during daily activities like eating, walking, or listening. The key is to be fully engaged in the here and now, observing your thoughts and sensations without getting caught up in them.

Meditation, on the other hand, is a more formal practice. It often involves setting aside time to sit in quiet reflection or concentration, focusing your attention to achieve a mentally clear and emotionally calm state. There are many forms of meditation, including mindfulness meditation, where the focus is on maintaining awareness of the present moment. Other forms include concentration meditation, which involves focusing on a single point (like a mantra, visual object, or the breath), and transcendental meditation, which involves repeating a specific mantra in a structured way.

In essence, while all mindfulness can be considered a form of meditation, not all meditation is specifically about mindfulness. Meditation is often a more structured practice used to train the mind and achieve specific states of consciousness, whereas mindfulness is a quality that can be brought to any moment in everyday life. Both practices complement each other and can lead to increased self-awareness, reduced stress, and a deeper sense of peace and well-being.

So, if you wanna look into meditation practices other than mindfulness, here's a good list to start:

1. Transcendental Meditation: Involves silently repeating a personal mantra in a specific way, promoting a state of relaxed awareness.

2. Guided Meditation: Uses verbal guidance from a teacher or a recording to lead you through a meditative experience, often

involving visualizing peaceful scenes or journeys.

3. Vipassana Meditation: An ancient Indian form of meditation that means to see things as they really are. It focuses on deep interconnection between mind and body, which can be experienced directly by disciplined attention to physical sensations.

4. Loving-kindness Meditation (Metta): Aims to cultivate an attitude of love and kindness toward everything, even a person's enemies and sources of stress.

5. Body Scan or Progressive Relaxation: Involves scanning your body for areas of tension and consciously releasing it.

6. Zen Meditation (Zazen): A form of seated meditation that is part of Buddhist practice, focusing on regulated breathing and posture with an emphasis on mindfulness.

Self-Compassion

Self-compassion is a powerful antidote to negative self-talk. It's about treating yourself with the same kindness, understanding, and support you'd offer a good friend. When you practice self-compassion, you recognize that being imperfect, making mistakes, and encountering life's challenges are all part of the shared human experience.

First, self-compassion involves self-kindness. This means being gentle and understanding with yourself, rather than harshly critical or judgmental. Imagine how you'd comfort a friend in a similar situation and apply that same empathy to yourself.

Second, self-compassion requires mindfulness. It's about being aware of your own suffering, recognizing it, but not over-identifying with it. This balance allows you to acknowledge your feelings without being swept up in them. It's about noticing your negative self-talk but not letting it define your self-worth.

Third, it includes a sense of common humanity. Often, negative self-talk isolates us. We think we're the only ones struggling or failing. Self-compassion reminds us that everyone makes mistakes and experiences hardship. You're not alone in your struggles.

Practicing self-compassion can be transformative, especially when combating negative self-talk. It shifts the narrative from one of isolation and self-critique to one of connectedness and self-care. This shift doesn't happen overnight, but with practice, it can significantly improve mental well-being, resilience, and overall happiness.

Remember, being compassionate to yourself is not about self-pity or laziness. It's about acknowledging your humanity, embracing your imperfections, and treating yourself with the same respect and kindness you would show others. It's a skill that, once learned, can change not only how you talk to yourself but also how you engage with the world.

Positive Self-Talk

Positive self-talk is an essential step in shifting our internal dialogue, but it's important to remember that simply telling ourselves we're fantastic can sometimes feel forced, almost as if we're not being truthful with ourselves. There's real value in tempering these affirmations to align more closely with what feels genuine to us. It's about finding phrases that resonate, that feel like something you can gradually grow into. For instance, saying to yourself, "I commit to loving myself a little more each day," or "I commit to doing my best each day," carries a sense of authenticity. It's about acknowledging progress, not perfection. Phrases like "I'm better than I was" can be incredibly empowering because they recognize improvement and personal growth.

Think of positive self-talk as a much-needed counterweight to the often overwhelming scale of negative self-talk. It's a well-established fact that our brains have a tendency towards a negativity bias, meaning we're naturally more inclined to pay attention to negative experiences than positive ones. Recognizing this, it becomes not just reasonable, but necessary, to consciously lean a bit more into positivity to strike a balance. This isn't about unrealistically painting everything with a rosy brush or denying the reality of challenges – it's about ensuring a fair and balanced internal dialogue. Imagine it as giving both sides of a debate an equal chance to be heard. It's not fair, nor is it productive, to constantly let the critical, doubting part of you dominate the conversation, while the supportive, affirmative side gets overlooked or silenced. Allowing yourself to engage in positive self-talk is like giving a voice to a friend who's been waiting patiently for their turn to speak. It's not about drowning out the negatives with relentless optimism, but about letting the positive aspects of yourself and your experiences have their rightful place at the table.

Accept the Basic Facts of Life

Much of the distress we experience in life often stems from a lack of awareness or acceptance of life's fundamental truths. For instance, say someone commits to never losing their temper. It's a common wish, yet it's an unrealistic expectation for any average person. Anger, like many other emotions, is a natural part of the human experience. By setting unattainable standards like never feeling angry, we set ourselves up for frustration and disappointment.

This scenario is just one among countless basic realities of life that, when not acknowledged or accepted, can lead to unnecessary suffering.

Understanding and accepting these simple truths can significantly reduce our emotional struggles and lead to a more balanced and fulfilling life.

Here are a handful of these truths:

1. Perfection is Unattainable: A common source of negative self-talk is the pursuit of perfection. Accept that mistakes and imperfections are part of being human. For instance, if you're berating yourself for not delivering a perfect presentation, remind yourself that it's okay not to be perfect. What matters is the effort and learning from the experience.

2. Failure is Inevitable: Often, we engage in negative self-talk after experiencing failure. It's essential to accept that failure is a natural part of life and growth. Every successful person has faced setbacks; what's important is how they used these experiences to improve.

3. Rejection is Not a Reflection of Your Worth: Whether it's a job, a relationship, or a social situation, rejection can lead to harsh self-criticism. Recognize that rejection is a universal

experience and doesn't define your value as a person.

4. Comparisons are Misleading: In the age of social media, it's easy to fall into the trap of comparing yourself to others. Accept that everyone's journey is different and that these comparisons often ignore the complex realities behind each person's life.

5. Control is Limited: Negative self-talk can arise when things don't go as planned. Understand that you can't control every aspect of life. Focus on your response to situations, rather than stressing over uncontrollable events.

6. Change is Constant: Fear of change can be a significant source of anxiety and negative self-talk. Embracing change as a natural and often positive part of life can help reduce this anxiety.

By accepting these basic facts, you can shift your internal dialogue from criticism and unrealistic expectations to one of understanding, resilience, and self-compassion.

Before We Get Started…

Remember, mindfulness journaling is a personal practice, and these questions are meant to guide and inspire you. Feel free to adapt and modify them to suit your needs and preferences. Explore, reflect, and embrace the opportunity to deepen your self-awareness and cultivate a sense of inner peace.

Date ___ / ___ / ___ : S   M   T   W   Th   F   S

I feel:
(please circle)

because   because   because   because   because
_____   _____   _____   _____   _____
_____   _____   _____   _____   _____

Today I Am Grateful For

1. _____
2. _____
3. _____

What could help transform today into a remarkable day?

Reflective Writing

What strategies can I use to increase positive self-talk?

_____

_____

_____

_____

_____

_____

_____

_____

Which of the following is an example of negative self-talk?

A) "I can handle this situation."

B) "I'll never be good enough."

C) "I am capable and confident."

D) "I am proud of my accomplishments."

All Are Correct - Choose The Response You Feel Is Most Important To Remember

Date ___ / ___ / ___ : S   M   T   W   Th   F   S

I feel:
(please circle)

because   because   because   because   because

_____ _____ _____ _____ _____

_____ _____ _____ _____ _____

Today I Am Grateful For

1. _____
2. _____
3. _____

What could help transform today into a remarkable day?

Reflective Writing

How can I become more aware of my negative self-talk?

_____

_____

_____

_____

_____

_____

_____

How can you combat negative self-talk?

A) By surrounding yourself with positive people.

B) By avoiding negative thoughts altogether.

C) By accepting that you will always have negative thoughts.

D) By constantly criticizing and berating yourself.

All Are Correct - Choose The Response You Feel Is Most Important To Remember

Date ___ / ___ / ___ : S   M   T   W   Th   F   S

I feel:
(please circle)

because   because   because   because   because
_____ _____ _____ _____ _____
_____ _____ _____ _____ _____

Today I Am Grateful For

1. _____
2. _____
3. _____

What could help transform today into a remarkable day?

Reflective Writing

What techniques can I use to combat negative
thoughts and feelings?

_____

_____

_____

_____

_____

_____

_____

_____

Which of the following is NOT a way to challenge negative self-talk?

A) Replacing negative thoughts with positive ones.

B) Recognizing and analyzing the evidence for and against the negative thought.

C) Engaging in self-care activities.

D) Ignoring and suppressing negative thoughts.

All Are Correct - Choose The Response You Feel Is Most Important To Remember

Date ___ / ___ / ___ : S M T W Th F S

I feel:
(please circle)

because _____ because _____ because _____ because _____ because _____

Today I Am Grateful For
1. _____
2. _____
3. _____

What could help transform today into a remarkable day?

Reflective Writing
How can I set realistic goals for myself to prevent negative self-talk?

_____
_____
_____
_____
_____
_____
_____

What is the first step to combating negative self-talk?

A) Understanding and acknowledging the negative thoughts.

B) Talking to a friend or loved one about your negative thoughts.

C) Distracting yourself from negative thoughts.

D) Believing that you are capable of overcoming negative self-talk.

All Are Correct - Choose The Response You Feel Is Most Important To Remember

Date ___ / ___ / ___ : S   M   T   W   Th   F   S

I feel:
(please circle)

because   because   because   because   because

_____ _____ _____ _____ _____

_____ _____ _____ _____ _____

Today I Am Grateful For

1. _____
2. _____
3. _____

What could help transform today into a remarkable day?

Reflective Writing

How can I use positive affirmations to combat negative self-talk?

_____

_____

_____

_____

_____

_____

_____

Which statement is an example of positive self-talk?

A) "I'll never be good enough."
B) "I am a failure."
C) "I am capable and resilient."
D) "I always mess everything up."

All Are Correct - Choose The Response You Feel Is Most Important To Remember

Date ___ / ___ / ___ : S   M   T   W   Th   F   S

I feel:
(please circle)

because   because   because   because   because
_____   _____   _____   _____   _____
_____   _____   _____   _____   _____

Today I Am Grateful For

1. _____
2. _____
3. _____

What could help transform today into a remarkable day?

Reflective Writing

How can I recognize and change my thinking
patterns to reduce negative self-talk?

_____

_____

_____

_____

_____

_____

_____

What is an important aspect of practicing positive self-talk?

A) Only focusing on your strengths and achievements.

B) Ignoring any negative thoughts or criticism.

C) Repeating positive affirmations that you don't truly believe.

D) Being honest and realistic with yourself.

All Are Correct - Choose The Response You Feel Is Most Important To Remember

Date ___ / ___ / ___ : S   M   T   W   Th   F   S

I feel:
(please circle)

because   because   because   because   because

_____ _____ _____ _____ _____

_____ _____ _____ _____ _____

Today I Am Grateful For

1. _____
2. _____
3. _____

What could help transform today into a remarkable day?

Reflective Writing

What techniques can I use to effectively counter
negative self-talk?

_____

_____

_____

_____

_____

_____

_____

Why is it important to challenge negative self-talk?

A) It can lead to increased confidence and self-esteem.

B) It can help you ignore any negative emotions.

C) It can make you more likable to others.

D) It can help you avoid facing your problems.

All Are Correct - Choose The Response You Feel Is Most Important To Remember

Date ___ / ___ / ___ : S   M   T   W   Th   F   S

I feel:
(please circle)

because   because   because   because   because

_____   _____   _____   _____   _____

_____   _____   _____   _____   _____

Today I Am Grateful For

1. _____
2. _____
3. _____

What could help transform today into a remarkable day?

Reflective Writing

What are some practical ways to stay motivated
and prevent negative self-talk?

_____

_____

_____

_____

_____

_____

_____

How can mindfulness practice help combat negative self-talk?

A) By distracting you from negative thoughts.

B) By suppressing negative thoughts.

C) By allowing you to observe and acknowledge your thoughts without judgment.

D) By forcing you to focus on your negative thoughts.

All Are Correct - Choose The Response You Feel Is Most Important To Remember

Date ___ / ___ / ___ : S   M   T   W   Th   F   S

I feel:
(please circle)

because   because   because   because   because
_____   _____   _____   _____   _____
_____   _____   _____   _____   _____

Today I Am Grateful For

1. _____
2. _____
3. _____

What could help transform today into a remarkable day?

Reflective Writing

How can I practice self-compassion to combat
negative self-talk?

_____

_____

_____

_____

_____

_____

_____

Which of the following is a sign that you are engaging in negative self-talk?

A) You make an effort to improve yourself.
B) You accept compliments from others.
C) You constantly criticize and belittle yourself.
D) You seek out positive experiences and relationships.

All Are Correct - Choose The Response You Feel Is Most Important To Remember

Date ___ / ___ / ___ : S   M   T   W   Th   F   S

I feel:
(please circle)

because   because   because   because   because
_____ _____ _____ _____ _____
_____ _____ _____ _____ _____

Today I Am Grateful For

1. _____
2. _____
3. _____

What could help transform today into a remarkable day?

Reflective Writing

What positive self-talk techniques can I use to help me
stay focused on my goals?

_____

_____

_____

_____

_____

_____

_____

How can seeking support from others help you combat negative self-talk?

A) Others can offer a different perspective and challenge your negative thoughts.

B) Others can distract you from your negative thoughts.

C) Others can make you feel worse about yourself.

D) Others can tell you what you want to hear.

All Are Correct - Choose The Response You Feel Is Most Important To Remember

Date ___ / ___ / ___: S M T W Th F S

I feel:
(please circle)

because because because because because
_____ _____ _____ _____ _____
_____ _____ _____ _____ _____

Today I Am Grateful For

1. _____
2. _____
3. _____

What could help transform today into a remarkable day?

Reflective Writing

How can I use mindfulness techniques to combat negative self-talk?

_____

_____

_____

_____

_____

_____

_____

Which statement is an example of negative self-talk?

A) "I am capable and valuable."
B) "I'll never be good enough for anyone."
C) "I am constantly improving."
D) "I am proud of my achievements."

All Are Correct - Choose The Response You Feel Is Most Important To Remember

Date ___ / ___ / ___ : S M T W Th F S

I feel:
(please circle)

because   because   because   because   because

_____ _____ _____ _____ _____

_____ _____ _____ _____ _____

Today I Am Grateful For

1. _____
2. _____
3. _____

What could help transform today into a remarkable day?

Reflective Writing
What techniques can I use to manage stress and prevent negative self-talk?

_____

_____

_____

_____

_____

_____

_____

_____

How can gratitude practice combat negative self-talk?

A) By making you realize that everyone has problems and struggles.

B) By forcing you to focus on the negative aspects of your life.

C) By making you feel guilty for having negative thoughts.

D) By making you appreciate the good things in your life.

All Are Correct - Choose The Response You Feel Is Most Important To Remember

Date ___ / ___ / ___ : S   M   T   W   Th   F   S

I feel:
(please circle)

because   because   because   because   because
_____ _____ _____ _____ _____
_____ _____ _____ _____ _____

Today I Am Grateful For
1. _____
2. _____
3. _____

What could help transform today into a remarkable day?

Reflective Writing
How can I use self-care to combat negative self-talk?

_____

_____

_____

_____

_____

_____

_____

_____

What is an important aspect of practicing self-compassion to combat negative self-talk?

A) Being critical of yourself and your mistakes.

B) Comparing yourself to others.

C) Being understanding and forgiving towards yourself.

D) Blaming and shaming yourself for your negative thoughts.

All Are Correct - Choose The Response You Feel Is Most Important To Remember

Date ___ / ___ / ___ : S   M   T   W   Th   F   S

I feel:
(please circle)

because   because   because   because   because
_____   _____   _____   _____   _____
_____   _____   _____   _____   _____

Today I Am Grateful For

1. _____
2. _____
3. _____

What could help transform today into a remarkable day?

Reflective Writing

What activities can I do to help me stay positive
and combat negative self-talk?

_____

_____

_____

_____

_____

_____

_____

What can happen if negative self-talk goes unchecked?

A) You may become overly confident.
B) You may believe everything you think.
C) You may become more self-aware.
D) You may experience low self-esteem and self-worth.

All Are Correct - Choose The Response You Feel Is Most Important To Remember

Date ___ / ___ / ___ : S M T W Th F S

I feel:
(please circle)

because   because   because   because   because
_____   _____   _____   _____   _____
_____   _____   _____   _____   _____

Today I Am Grateful For

1. _____
2. _____
3. _____

What could help transform today into a remarkable day?

Reflective Writing

How can I use positive self-talk to build
confidence and self-esteem?

_____

_____

_____

_____

_____

_____

_____

Which of the following is NOT a common type of negative self-talk?

A) Catastrophizing
B) Personalizing
C) Rationalizing
D) Comparing

All Are Correct - Choose The Response You Feel Is Most Important To Remember

As we reach the final pages of this journey through "Positive Mindset," I want to extend my heartfelt thanks to you. Your commitment to exploring positivity and its transformative power is not only commendable but a testament to your desire for personal growth and a richer, more fulfilling life experience.

Remember, the journey towards a positive mindset is ongoing and ever-evolving. Each day presents new opportunities to apply these principles, to learn, and to grow. I encourage you to revisit these pages whenever you need a reminder of your incredible potential to foster positivity and resilience in the face of life's challenges.

As we part ways, I leave you with a quote that has been a guiding star in my journey: "The greatest discovery of any generation is that a human can alter his life by altering his attitude."

— William James.

Thank you for allowing me to be a part of your journey. May your path be filled with light, hope, and endless possibilities. Farewell, and may you carry the spirit of positivity with you, today and always.

With gratitude and best wishes,

Sensei Paul David

Reflective Writing

The End

As you close the pages of this mindfulness journal, remember that each word you've written is a step on your journey towards self-awareness and inner peace. Embrace the moments of clarity, the revelations, and even the uncertainties you've encountered along the way. Let this journal be a testament to your growth and a reminder that every day offers a new opportunity to be present, to observe, and to appreciate the simple wonders of life. Carry these lessons forward, and may your path be filled with mindful moments and serene reflections. Until we meet again in these pages, be gentle with yourself and stay anchored in the now.

Mindfulness isn't difficult, we just need to remember to do it.

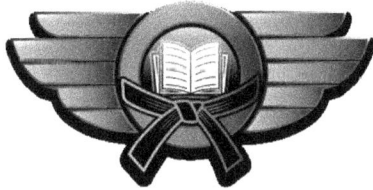

Thank You!

If you found this book helpful, I would be grateful if you would **post an honest review on Amazon** so this book can reach other supportive readers like you!

All you need to do is digitally flip to the back and leave your review. Or visit amazon.com/author/senseipauldavid click the correct book cover and click on the blue link next to the yellow stars that say, "customer reviews."

As always...
It's a great day to be alive!

Get/Share Your FREE SSD Mental Health Chronicles at
www.senseiselfdevelopment.care

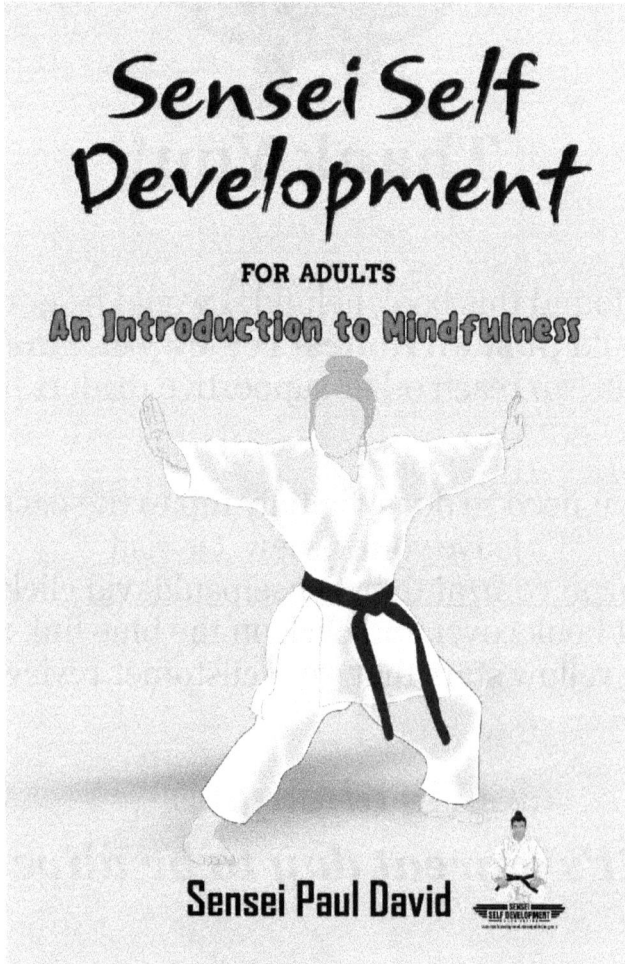

Sensei Self Development

FOR ADULTS

An Introduction to Mindfulness

Sensei Paul David

Check Out The SSD Chronicles
Series <u>CLICK HERE</u>

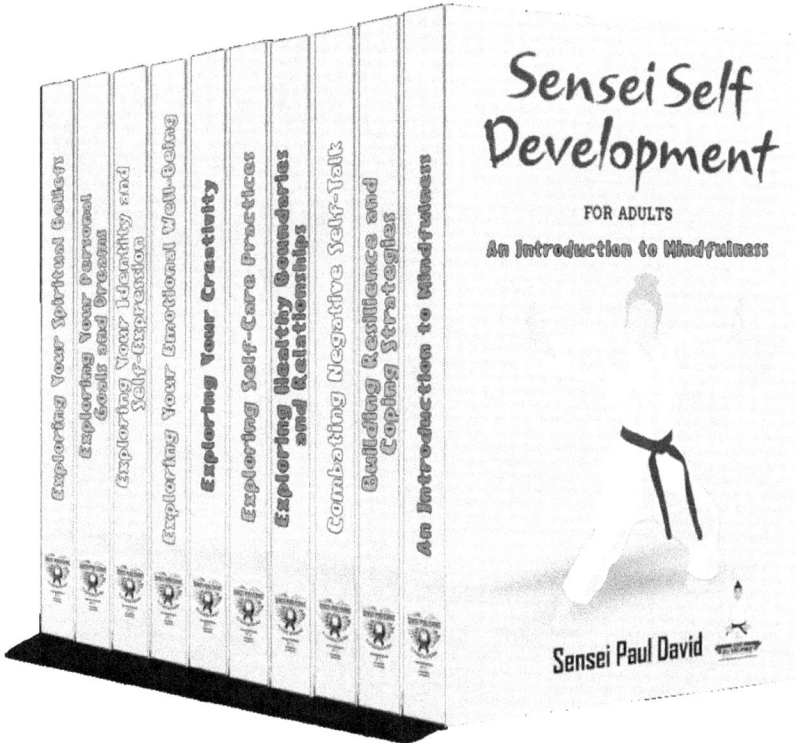

Get/Share Your FREE All-Ages Mental Health eBook Now at

www.senseiselfdevelopment.com

Or CLICK HERE

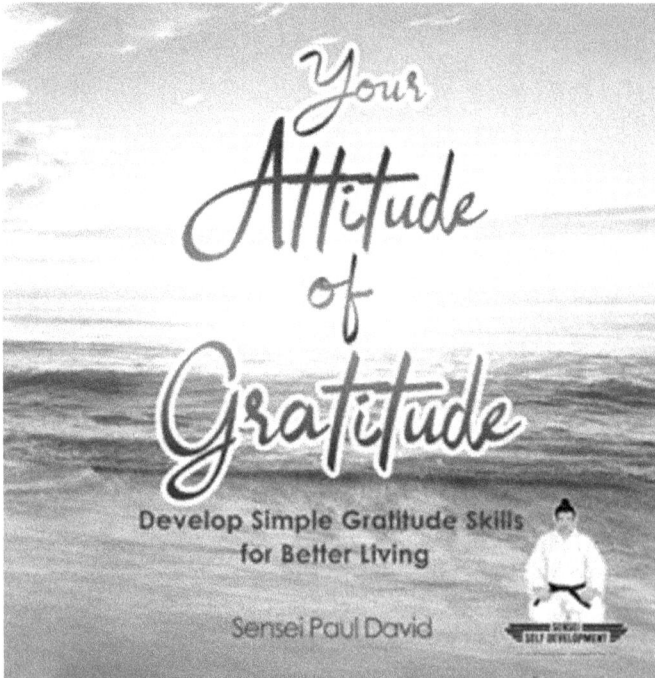

senseiselfdevelopment.com

Click Another Book In The SSD BOOK SERIES:

senseipublishing.com/SSD_SERIES

CLICK HERE

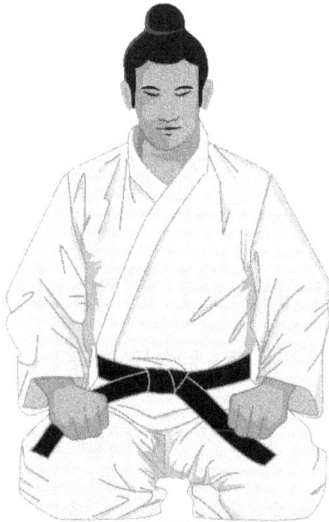

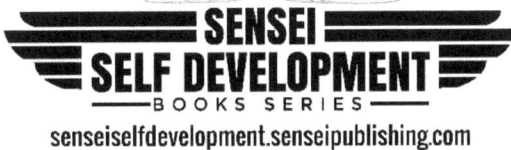

senseiselfdevelopment.senseipublishing.com

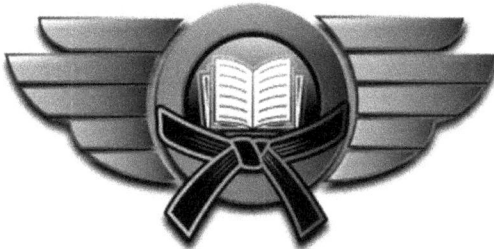

Join Our Publishing Journey!

If you would like to receive FREE BOOKS, please visit **www.senseipublishing.com**. Join our newsletter by entering your email address in the pop-up box

Follow Sensei Paul David on Amazon

CLICK THE LOGO BELOW

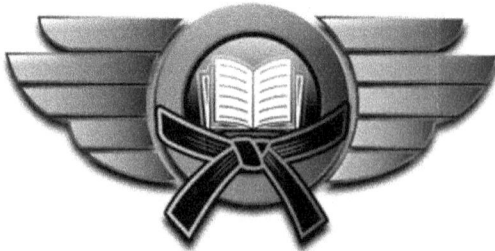

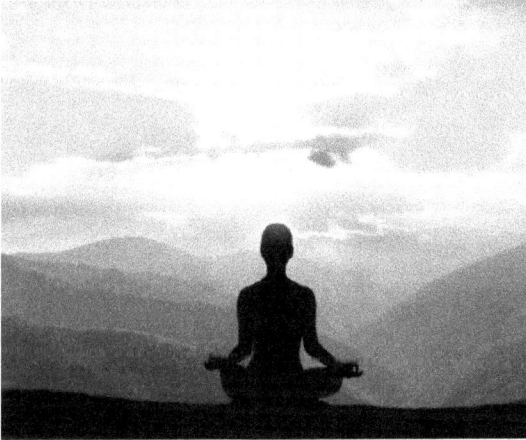

FREE BONUS!!!
Experience Over 25 FREE Engaging Guided Meditations!

Prized Skills & Practices for Adults & Kids. Help Restore Deep-Sleep, Lower Stress, Improve Posture, Navigate Uncertainty & More.

Download the Free Insight Timer App and click the link below:
http://insig.ht/sensei_paul

About Sensei Publishing

Sensei Publishing commits itself to helping people of all ages transform into better versions of themselves by providing high-quality and research-based self-development books with an emphasis on mental health and guided meditations. Sensei Publishing offers well-written e-books, audiobooks, paperbacks and online courses that simplify complicated but practical topics in line with its mission to inspire people towards positive transformation.

It's a great day to be alive!

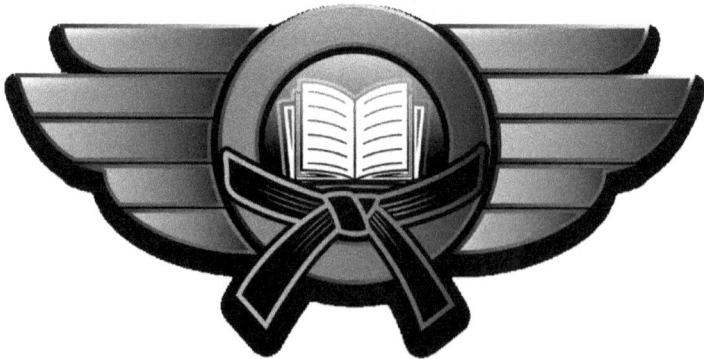

About the Author

I create simple & transformative eBooks & Guided Meditations for Adults & Children proven to help navigate uncertainty, solve niche problems & bring families closer together.

I'm a former finance project manager, private pilot, jiu-jitsu instructor, musician & former University of Toronto Fitness Trainer. I prefer a science-based approach to focus on these & other areas in my life to stay humble & hungry to evolve. I hope you enjoy my work and I'd love to hear your feedback.

- It's a great day to be alive!

Sensei Paul David

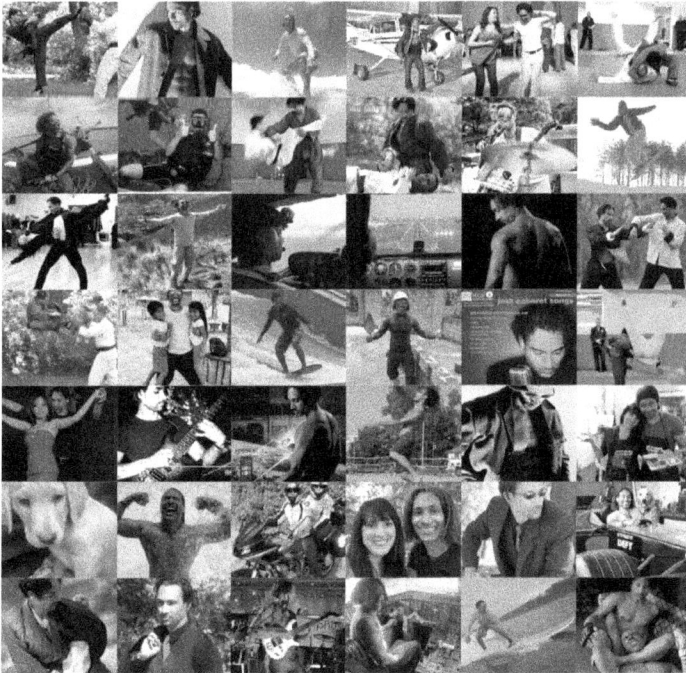

Scan & Follow/Like/Subscribe: Facebook, Instagram, YouTube: @senseipublishing

Scan using your phone/iPad camera for Social Media
Visit us at www.senseipublishing.com and sign up for our
newsletter to learn more about our exciting books and to
experience our FREE Guided Meditations for Kids & Adults.